HERBAL
BEAUTY

Caleb Warnock &
Kirsten Skirvin

DISCOVER THE LONG-LOST SKILLS OF SELF-RELIANCE

My name is Caleb Warnock, and I've been working for years to learn how to return to forgotten skills, the skills of our ancestors. As our world becomes increasingly unstable, self-reliance becomes invaluable. Throughout this series, *The Backyard Renaissance*, I will share with you the lost skills of self-sufficiency and healthy living. Come with me and other do-it-yourself experimenters, and rediscover the joys and success of simple self-reliance.

FAMILIUS

Published by Familius LLC, www.familius.com

Familius books are available at special discounts for bulk purchases for sales promotions or for family or corporate use. Special editions, including personalized covers, excerpts of existing books, or books with corporate logos, can be created in large quantities for special needs. For more information, contact Premium Sales at 559-876-2170 or email orders@familius.com.

Library of Congress Cataloging-in-Publication Data
2015956718

ISBN: 9781942934523
eISBN: 9781944822354

Printed in the United States of America

Edited by Liza Hagerman
Cover design by David Miles
Book design by David Miles and Brooke Jorden

10 9 8 7 6 5 4 3 2 1
First Edition

CONTENTS

INTRODUCTION xiii

FACIAL TREATMENTS 1

ROSE WATER SPRITZER 1

ESSENTIAL OIL ROSE WATER SPRITZ 3

HORSE CHESTNUT-INFUSED OIL FOR WRINKLES........ 4

HORSE CHESTNUT-INFUSED OIL MAKEUP
    REMOVER.. 6

OLIVE OIL FACIAL CLEANSER 7

KIRSTEN'S FILLY FACE CREAM 7

CHICKWEED-INFUSED OIL................................. 9

HONEY JOJOBA FACIAL SCRUB AND ACNE
    TREATMENT..10

CLAY MASK 11

COSMETICS 13

ALL-NATURAL BLUSH 13

ALL-NATURAL RED LIP STAIN 14

TEETH WHITENING SOLUTION 16

DEODORANTS, LOTIONS, AND SALVES 19

ARIZONA HEAT HOMEMADE DEODORANT 19

ARIZONA HEAT HOMEMADE DEODORANT FOR
SENSITIVE SKIN 20

CALENDULA- OR COMFREY-INFUSED OIL 22

COMFREY SALVE 22

ACNE SALVE 23

ECZEMA SKIN TREATMENTS 25

ECZEMA SALVE 26

ECZEMA TEA 27

ECZEMA CREAM 28

THE "NO POO" SHAMPOO REVOLUTION .. 31

BAKING SODA WET SHAMPOO 33

ARROWROOT DRY SHAMPOO 33

HONEY WET SHAMPOO FOR NORMAL HAIR 34

HONEY WET SHAMPOO FOR OILY HAIR 35

HONEY FRANKINCENSE SHAMPOO 36

TWO-PART NATURAL BORAX SHAMPOO 36

YUCCA ROOT POWDER SHAMPOO 38

YUCCA LEAF OR ROOT SHAMPOO 38

CONDITIONER AND HAIR STYLING 41

APPLE CIDER VINEGAR CONDITIONER &
DETANGLER SPRITZ 41

DEEP CONDITIONER 42

HOMEMADE HAIRSPRAY 43

HOMEMADE HAIR MOUSSE 44

"NEVER SNOTTY" HAIR GEL 45

HARD LESSON LEARNED 47

AVOIDING TOXIC SHOCK SYNDROME WITH MENSTRUAL CUPS 51

AND FOR FUN . . . TWO HISTORIC COMPLEXION REMEDIES 55

A s we learn about the chemicals in our diets, cosmetics, hygiene products, and pharmaceuticals, many of us have become determined to distance ourselves from their potentially harmful side effects. Are all these chemicals really necessary? Do their manufacturers have our safety first in mind—or their profits? Are there natural alternatives that might even help us save money? In this book, you will find 100 percent natural and homemade substitutes for deodorant, hairspray, lotion, fragrance, wrinkle cream, eczema and acne treatments, teeth whitening, makeup remover, and facial cleanser and many options for all-natural, homemade shampoos, hair conditioner, and even hair detangler. You'll also find critical information about—and ways to prevent—toxic shock syndrome. Starting today, you can easily and inexpensively remove unnecessary chemicals and health risks from your daily life. Take control of your health and future using time-tested natural solutions.

Disclaimer: Kirsten Skirvin and Caleb Warnock are not medical doctors. This book presents time-honored historic herbal and natural methods, but this information is not medical advice and should not be treated as such. The herbal products and methods identified in this book have not been evaluated by the FDA and are not intended to treat or prevent disease. The information provided here is for educational purposes only. You should research and make your own decisions about your health.

In this book, you will find a discussion of conditions these products have been used to aid. We are not claiming that the product will cure any of these diseases or that we created them to cure these diseases. We are merely reporting that people have used the products to aid these conditions. Always seek the advice of your physician or a licensed medical professional for diagnosis and treatment of any and all medical conditions.

INTRODUCTION:
A DILIGENT SEEKER OF A
CHEMICAL-FREE LIFE

My name is Kirsten, pronounced *Kear-sten*. Probably due to bluntly correcting and defending the pronunciation of my name since I could speak, I grew up a bit of a tomboy. My first experience with makeup was my junior Christmas formal. My older sister and my mother held me down while they applied mascara (a horrible experience) and other items to make me "beautiful." I felt like I had spiders on my eyes—and I am beyond terrified of spiders. When I finally decided to marry, one of my biggest qualifications was whether my future husband could beat me at arm wrestling. Needless to say, beauty techniques were far from my mind. Well, he won at arm wrestling, and seven children later, I decided maybe I ought to pay more attention to all the advertisements for beautifying aging women. I enthusiastically invested more money than I care to admit on magical serums to make me beautiful. Surprisingly, I still looked like me—which I decided was just fine.

After earning a Master Herbalist certification, I began to read the labels of all the products that I owned. Wow! That very long, unpronounceable word and chemical was touching my skin? My face? My lips? For years, I decided there was no way to get around it, but on a family vacation, my sister-in-law told me about how washing her face with oil had cleared up her acne. I was shocked and excited! There was a way out of chemicals and overpriced products—which I never used anyway because they took too much time and I was afraid of running out and having to buy more. Was that hassle logical? No. I became a diligent seeker of a no-chemical life.

Now, in the spirit of full disclosure, I admit that I sometimes lose all of my common sense and purchase a wonderful "something" guaranteed to keep me young, vibrant, etc. I get caught up in the promises and testimonials, and then the product sits in my drawer, barely used.

My hope for you is that you will use these simple recipes to enhance your natural beauty. Add, mix, and change the recipes as you see fit and according to your individual needs. Learn from your mistakes, as I have (my sister can attest to this), and never be afraid to try something new.

KIRSTEN SKIRVIN, NOVEMBER 2015

FACIAL TREATMENTS

ROSE WATER SPRITZER

For this recipe, you may use petals from roses of any color, and they may be wild or cultivated. If you want your rose water to be rose scented, you will need to use roses that have a natural fragrance. Do not mix different types of roses because they have different smells that may not be pleasing when combined. Mixing rose petal colors can also result in off rose water colors.

Fresh rose petals (enough to pack into a jar)   **Distilled water**

 Rinse the rose petals in cold water (sometimes roses have aphids). Pack the petals into a glass mason jar of any size.

2   Pour just enough distilled water into the mason jar to cover the rose petals. Put a lid on the jar.

3   Put the mason jar in a saucepan. Fill the pan halfway with tap water. To protect the glass jar from the direct heat at the bottom of the pan, put an upturned quart jar lid at the bottom of the pan, between the pan and the jar. Turn the heat on low and simmer the jar for 20 minutes. Remove from heat.

4   Strain the liquid from the rose petals using a mesh strainer, reusable straining cloth (available at SeedRenaissance.com), or cheesecloth. If you want your rose water to have a stronger fragrance, proceed to Step 5.

5   Repeat Steps 1–4 with fresh rose petals, but use the finished rose water instead of new distilled water each time. The strongest scent is achieved if you reuse the rose water 3–4 times total. Store the rose water in a lidded container.

Tip: You can also use other flower petals, lemongrass, or other strongly scented herbs to make a spritzer. Explore and have fun creating scents!

ESSENTIAL OIL ROSE WATER SPRITZ

Some people find it more convenient to make their rose water from commercially prepared essential oil instead of gathering rose petals. The good news is that it takes very little oil to make a cup of rose water. Although this recipe is for rose water, you can substitute any essential oil that you want.

1 cup hot water

1 drop rose essential oil (or essential oil of your choice)

1. Pour water into a spritzer bottle. Add essential oil.

2. Close the bottle tightly and shake before using.

3. If your spritz isn't strongly fragranced enough, add one more drop, shake, and try again. Some people prefer to use several drops, and essential oil strength varies widely depending on how much "carrier oil" is used in the formulation. (Even so-called "pure" essential oils often contain carrier oils.)

HORSE CHESTNUT-INFUSED OIL FOR WRINKLES

Horse chestnuts (scientific name Aesculus hippocastanum) reportedly contain a beneficial substance called aescin, which is a phytochemical (meaning it is biologically active) known to help tone skin, reduce the appearance of veins, and reduce wrinkles. The infused oil of chestnuts is widely available online and in health food stores, but you can also make your own if you have access to a chestnut tree or can purchase fresh chestnuts.

An oil infusion simply means you put the chestnuts in oil for a time, so that it can leach the beneficial phytochemicals from the nuts and shells, and then remove the nuts and shells and use the oil. There are two methods for making an infused oil; choose the method below that fits your time frame.

Horse chestnuts   **Olive oil**

METHOD #1 (SLOW METHOD)

Crack the shells of the chestnuts, remove and discard the shells, and put the nuts in a glass mason jar. (Use a hammer to crack the shells, because they can be very tough.) Add enough olive oil to just cover the nuts.

2   Cover the jar and shake it once a day for two weeks.

3   After two weeks, remove the nuts and strain the oil
    with a reusable straining cloth (available at SeedRe-
    naissance.com) or cheesecloth. Store the oil in a
    lidded jar for up to a year in a cool, dry, dark place.

METHOD #2 (FAST METHOD)

1   Crack the shells of the chestnuts, remove and
    discard the shells, and put the nuts in a glass mason
    jar. (Use a hammer to crack the shells, because they
    can be very tough.) Add enough olive oil to just cover
    the nuts. Cover the jar.

2   Put the jar in a saucepan of water on the stove.
    To protect the glass jar from the direct heat at the
    bottom of the pan, put an upturned quart jar lid at
    the bottom of the pan, between the pan and the
    jar. Simmer the jar until the temperature of the oil
    reaches 95 degrees, then turn off the heat.

3   Rewarm the oil to 95 degrees four or five more times
    over the next 24 hours. Be sure to keep the tempera-
    ture of the oil in the jar below 100 degrees, because

temperatures over 100 degrees can begin to damage the phytochemicals in the chestnuts.

 Strain the oil with a reusable straining cloth (available at SeedRenaissance.com) or cheesecloth. Store the oil in a lidded jar for up to a year in a cool, dry, dark place.

HORSE CHESTNUT-INFUSED OIL MAKEUP REMOVER

Horse chestnut oil can also be used as a makeup remover. "Not only does it clean off your makeup, it also cleans your face, and the olive oil is nutritive and healthy for your skin," Kirsten says. "This is also good because it will not irritate your skin or cause acne."

1–2 teaspoons Horse Chestnut-Infused Oil (see page 4)

1 Apply the oil to your face like a face cream.

2 Soak a washcloth in hot water and scrub your face with it in a circular motion.

OLIVE OIL FACIAL CLEANSER

Plain olive oil makes a great face cleanser. You can do this in the morning, at night, or both.

1-2 teaspoons olive Oil

1. Apply the oil to your face, rubbing in a circular motion.

2. Remove with very warm water and a washcloth.

KIRSTEN'S FILLY FACE CREAM

This cream is a favorite of Kirsten's and everyone she shares it with. She calls this "filly cream" (after a filly horse) because it is made with homemade Horse Chestnut–Infused Oil and because it makes her feel young. The citric acid in this recipe contains vitamin C and a preservative, which is good for your face.

2/3 cup rose water or distilled water

1/3 cup apricot oil

1/3 cup aloe vera

1/2 cup Horse Chestnut–Infused Oil (see page 4)

1/4 cup jojoba oil

2 tablespoons lecithin

1/2 ounce beeswax*

1 teaspoon citric acid

1 teaspoon lanolin**

2–3 drops lavender oil or other essential oil (for fragrance)

*When working with beeswax, it is important to remember that even small amounts never completely come off pans. For this reason, use a pan that will be dedicated to making only beeswax products, or use a clean pan from a thrift store.

**Lanolin is a natural emollient produced by sheep on their wool. Some lanolin products that are labeled "pure" may have ingredients added. Check the label, and if there are extra ingredients, consider purchasing different lanolin.

Tip: Some beeswax can be bought in pellets instead of chunks, which are easier to measure.

Caution: Many times, commercially processed and pelleted beeswax can have a smoky smell, which means that it was processed at too high a heat and the wax has been damaged. Do not use beeswax with a smoky smell, and do not use damaged beeswax in homemade beauty products.

1   Combine all ingredients in a quart glass mason jar.

2   Put the mason jar in a saucepan. Fill the pan halfway with tap water. To protect the glass jar from the direct heat at the bottom of the pan, put an upturned quart jar lid at the bottom of the pan, between the pan and the jar. Simmer the jar until the beeswax is completely melted.

3   Remove from heat. Whisk until creamy and ingredients are completely incorporated. A hand blender is ideal for this step.

4   Let cool until the face cream can be handled. Using a spatula, move the face cream to a clean jar or storage container with a lid. Use within 60 days.

CHICKWEED-INFUSED OIL

If you suffer from red blotches or unwanted rosy cheeks, using chickweed-infused oil can reduce the redness and heal your skin over time. Common chickweed is known scientifically as Stellaria media. Chickweed-infused oil is prepared like the chestnut oil infusion mentioned earlier in this book, but chickweed is always dried before being used to make an infusion because, due to their water content, green herbs can cause infused oil to grow bacteria or spoil. Chickweed can be harvested from the wild or from your garden if you are an experienced herbalist, or you can purchase dried chickweed online and at many health food stores.

1 ounce dried chickweed to every 4 ounces oil   **Olive oil**

1 To create the infusion, follow one of the two methods for Horse Chestnut–Infused Oil for Wrinkles (see page 4), substituting chickweed for the horse chestnuts. When making the chickweed-infused oil, you can also use jojoba oil instead of olive oil or use a mixture of half of each oil.

2 Apply the finished oil to your trouble areas with an applicator or your fingers. Let it stay on the skin for one minute, then wash it off with a very warm washcloth. If you are applying with your fingers, make

sure your fingers are clean and avoid putting your fingers back in the oil after touching your face. It is important to keep the oil sanitary.

CLAY MASK

You can achieve deep facial cleansing simply by using a clay mask. Kirsten recommends a bentonite clay mask available at health food stores.

Clay mask kit   *Water*

1   Mix the clay with the water and apply it to your face in a thin layer.

2   Leave the mask on for 15–20 minutes, then remove it by washing it off with a clean, warm washcloth.

HONEY JOJOBA FACIAL SCRUB AND ACNE TREATMENT

This scrub is used to gently exfoliate your skin. The honey and salt combine to act as a cleanser, and the jojoba oil softens, smooths, and protects the skin. The salt can be a little drying to the skin, but the jojoba counteracts that.

2 tablespoons honey
1 teaspoon salt

1/2 teaspoon jojoba oil

1. Stir ingredients together in a container that can be closed with a lid. Stir until completely incorporated, with the salt spread throughout the mixture.

2. Apply the scrub to your face, gently scrubbing in a circular motion, and then wash it off with a very warm washcloth.

3. Use this facial scrub once a week or as needed. It does not need to be refrigerated if used within a month.

Tip: Over time, the mixture may need to be stirred again before use, because the salt tends to settle and separate from the honey mixture.

COSMETICS

ALL-NATURAL BLUSH

People spend a lot of money on cosmetics, but there are all-natural, simple alternatives. This is one of those. To make homemade blush, all you need is beetroot powder, which you can find online and in health food stores. To make homemade beetroot powder, you will need the best-quality red beets.

1 red beet

1. Wash the beets carefully and slice them as thinly as possible. Allow them to to air-dry over many days, or dry them in a dehydrator.

2. Crush the dried beet slices with a hammer by placing them in a plastic zipper bag that can be

discarded afterward. Smash the bagged slices with the hammer until they are broken into pieces.

3

Put the pieces into a blender or food processor and pulse them to pulverize them more. It may not be possible to pulverize all of the dried beet pieces, but you should be able to sift out enough powder to use for making the homemade blush. Do not overtax your blender or food processor when trying to pulverize dried beets, because overworking the machine can cause permanent damage.

4

Brush or rub the naturally red powder onto your cheeks.

If you want your blush to be a little creamier, add a touch of Kirsten's Filly Face Cream (see page 8). If you want your blush to be a lighter color, add a touch of arrowroot powder.

ALL-NATURAL RED LIP STAIN

Not only is lipstick expensive, but Kirsten is concerned about the ingredients in typical purchased lipsticks because the product often ends up in your mouth—bringing with it ingredients that may not be safe for ingestion. "If you don't want to end up eating it, you probably shouldn't put it on your lips," she says. But all of the ingredients in this easy recipe are 100 percent natural and edible.

1 teaspoon beetroot powder   **Arrowroot powder (optional)**
Drops of vegetable glycerin*

*Glycerin, also spelled glycerine or glycerol, is a natural, odorless, colorless liquid derived from palm trees and soybeans. It is slightly sweet in flavor and is nontoxic. Glycerin is widely used in foods, candy, pharmaceuticals, and cosmetics. However, there are also synthetic glycerins sold that are derived from petroleum. Make sure when purchasing glycerin (available at any drugstore) that the label says it is vegetable glycerin, because synthetic glycerin can contain trace amounts of petroleum derivatives and processing chemicals that should not be used on the skin.

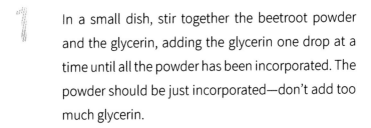

1   In a small dish, stir together the beetroot powder and the glycerin, adding the glycerin one drop at a time until all the powder has been incorporated. The powder should be just incorporated—don't add too much glycerin.

2   If the lip stain is redder than you like, add tiny amounts of arrowroot powder to lighten the shade of red until you have achieved a custom color that you love.

3 Store the lip stain in a small lidded container, which is available at health food stores and online. Lip stain can be applied with a lip brush. Reapply as needed.

Tip: You can add a tiny amount of beeswax to this recipe to make lipstick. Heat the lip stain to incorporate the beeswax, and pour the mixture into a blank lipstick container (sold online and at health food stores). However, because of the small amounts this recipe calls for, you may want to increase the amounts of the ingredients to make a larger batch.

Tip: You can also try staining your lips with the natural red juice of a beet. If the color is too red, you can add tiny amounts of arrowroot powder to the beet to lighten the shade before you apply it.

TEETH WHITENING SOLUTION

Both Caleb and Kirsten use natural hydrogen peroxide to whiten their teeth. Kirsten turned to this natural alternative after spending $300 to have her teeth professionally whitened by a dentist who created a custom dental tray for her to use at home with a commercial whitening solution—only to have her gums turn painfully red and swell. "I stopped and haven't used it since," she says. "I swish hydrogen peroxide in my mouth, and I have nice white teeth."

1 tablespoon hydrogen peroxide

 Swish the hydrogen peroxide in your mouth for 1–3 minutes, then spit it out. This whitens all of your teeth, does not make the teeth chalky, and is healthy for your gums. Hydrogen peroxide is also used to help remove dead skin cells and clean mouth lacerations.

DEODORANTS, LOTIONS, AND SALVES

ARIZONA HEAT HOMEMADE DEODORANT

"I lived in Arizona," says Kirsten. "Do you know how hot Arizona is? I have been using this homemade deodorant for five years and it works, even in the heat of the Southwest. I am living proof that you can make it through an Arizona summer with just this as your deodorant."

Tip: If you are working outside and it is over 100 degrees, reapplication may be necessary.

1/2 cup baking soda
1/2 cup cornstarch

Coconut oil or olive oil

1. Whisk the baking soda and cornstarch together in a bowl to sift them, creating a smooth, even mixture.

2. Stir in a drizzle of coconut oil and continue adding the oil several drops at a time until the mixture is creamy and smooth. Store in a lidded container.

3. Apply to your underarms as needed. This deodorant will store at room temperature for at least a month, but discard it if discoloration or a rancid odor develops.

FOR A GREAT BODY LOTION, USE JUST PLAIN COCONUT OIL. IT IS USED BY MANY MASSAGE THERAPISTS AND WAS RECOMMENDED TO KIRSTEN BY HER DOCTOR. HOWEVER, AVOID USING IT ON THE FACE BECAUSE THE PORES ARE SENSITIVE AND ARE PRONE TO CLOG, RESULTING IN ACNE. INSTEAD, USE OLIVE OIL ON THE FACE. OLIVE OIL ALSO NOURISHES AND MOISTURIZES THE SKIN AS IT IS ABSORBED. FOR INSTRUCTIONS ON MAKING ALL-NATURAL LOTION BARS, SEE THE BOOK *MAKE YOUR OWN HARD LOTION* BY CALEB WARNOCK AND AMBERLEE RYNN (SANGER, CA: FAMILIUS, 2015).

ARIZONA HEAT HOMEMADE DEODORANT FOR SENSITIVE SKIN

In classes that we have taught, some students have said that inexpensive baking soda gives them rashes, but they solved the problem by using baking soda in smaller amounts. With that in mind, we offer this second recipe for people who may have sensitive skin.

1 tablespoon baking soda (students preferred the Bob's Red Mill brand)

1/2 cup tapioca starch
Olive oil

1. Whisk the baking soda and tapioca starch together in a bowl to sift them, creating a smooth, even mixture.

2. Stir in a drizzle of olive oil and continue adding oil several drops at a time until the mixture is creamy and smooth. Store in a lidded container.

3. Apply to your underarms as needed. This deodorant will store at room temperature for at least a month, but discard it if discoloration or a rancid odor develops.

CALENDULA- OR COMFREY-INFUSED OIL

"Some people have chapped hands and need a little more help,"
says Kirsten. Comfrey-infused oil makes a really good salve or lotion.
Calendula creams and calendula-infused oils also work well.

Calendula petals or comfrey   **Olive oil**
  leaves

 To make your own calendula- or comfrey-infused oil, follow the instructions for one of the two recipes for Horse Chestnut–Infused Oil for Wrinkles (see page 4), substituting calendula petals or comfrey leaves for the chestnuts.

Tip: Be sure to use only dried comfrey leaves or dried calendula petals. If you want to add these plants to your herb garden, seeds for true comfrey and true medicinal, high-resin calendula are available at SeedRenaissance.com.

COMFREY SALVE

Comfrey is one of the largest herbs in the garden, with leaves that can be more than two feet long. Seeds are available at SeedRenaissance.com.

4 ounces Comfrey-Infused Oil   1 ounce beeswax*
   (see page 22)

*When working with beeswax, it is important to remember that even small amounts never completely come off pans. For this reason, use a pan that will be dedicated to making only beeswax products, or use a clean pan from a thrift store.

1   Melt both ingredients together in a saucepan over low heat. Stir to blend.

2   Pour into clean salve jars to cool.

Tip: Small salve jars are sold at health food stores.

ACNE SALVE

Perhaps the best all-natural acne treatment in the world is simply applying comfrey-infused olive oil to the face.

1–2 teaspoons Comfrey-Infused Oil (see page 22)

1 Leave the oil on your face for 1–2 minutes.

2 Wash it off with a very warm washcloth.

ECƷEMA SKIN TREATMENTS

A ccording to the National Eczema Association, eczema is a rash of the skin that cannot be cured but can be managed with good skin care. More than 30 million Americans suffer from this skin condition, which doctors call "atopic dermatitis."[1] Kirsten's niece and Caleb both suffer from eczema, but they have been able to control it with herbal skin treatments. "Chickweed does work great for eczema," says Kirsten. This book offers three eczema treatments, each based on chickweed. Common chickweed is known scientifically as *Stellaria media* and grows wild as a weed in many places, and it can be grown in a garden (seeds available at SeedRenaissance.com) or purchased as a dried herb.

ECZEMA SALVE

Chickweed is always dried before being used to make an oil infusion because, due to their water content, green herbs can cause infused oil to grow bacteria or spoil. To create the oil infusion needed for this recipe, follow one of the two recipes for Horse Chestnut–Infused Oil for Wrinkles (see page 4).

3 ounces Chickweed-Infused Oil (see page 10)

1 ounce beeswax*
1 ounce lanolin**

*When working with beeswax, it is important to remember that even small amounts never completely come off pans. For this reason, use a pan that will be dedicated to making only beeswax products, or use a clean pan from a thrift store.

**Lanolin is a natural emollient produced by sheep on their wool. Some lanolin products that are labeled "pure" may have ingredients added. Check the label, and if there are extra ingredients, consider purchasing different lanolin.

Tip: Some beeswax can be bought in pellets instead of chunks, which is easier to measure.

Caution: Many times, commercially processed and pelleted beeswax can have a smoky smell, which means that it was processed at too high a heat and the wax has been damaged. Do not buy beeswax with a smoky smell, and do not use damaged beeswax in homemade beauty products.

 Combine all ingredients in a quart glass mason jar.

 Put the mason jar in a saucepan. Fill the pan halfway with tap water. To protect the glass jar from the direct heat at the bottom of the pan, put an upturned quart jar lid at the bottom of the pan between the pan and the jar. Simmer the jar until the beeswax is completely melted.

 Remove from heat. Whisk until creamy and ingredients are completely incorporated. Let cool until the salve can be handled.

 Using a spatula, move the eczema salve to a clean jar or storage container with a lid. Use within 60 days.

ECZEMA TEA

Chickweed can also be taken internally as a tea.

1 teaspoon dried chickweed   **1 cup hot water**

1   Soak the dried herb in the tea for several minutes until the tea turns a pale green color.

2   Strain out the chickweed and drink the tea warm, or add it to a green smoothie.

3   Drink once a day for several weeks until you see an improvement in your eczema. Continue drinking the tea every few days to maintain the improved skin condition.

ECZEMA CREAM

Instead of creating a salve, which is thickened with beeswax, you can also create a cream to treat eczema.

2/3 cup rose water or distilled water

1/3 cup apricot oil

1/3 cup aloe vera

1/2 cup Chickweed-Infused Oil (see page 10)

1/4 cup jojoba oil

2 tablespoons lecithin

1/2 ounce beeswax*

1 teaspoon citric acid

1 teaspoon lanolin**

2–3 drops lavender oil or other essential oil (for fragrance)

When working with beeswax, it is important to remember that even small amounts never completely come off pans. For this reason, use a pan that will be dedicated to making only beeswax products, or use a clean pan from a thrift store.

**Lanolin is a natural emollient produced by sheep on their wool. Some lanolin products that are labeled "pure" may have ingredients added. Check the label, and if there are extra ingredients, consider purchasing different lanolin.*

Tip: Some beeswax can be bought in pellets instead of chunks, which are easier to measure.

Caution: Many times, commercially processed and pelleted beeswax can have a smoky smell, which means that it was processed at too high a heat and the wax has been damaged. Do not use beeswax with a smoky smell, and do not use damaged beeswax in homemade beauty products.

1   Combine all ingredients in a quart glass mason jar.

2   Put the mason jar in a saucepan. Fill the pan halfway with tap water. To protect the glass jar from the direct

heat at the bottom of the pan, put an upturned quart jar lid at the bottom of the pan, between the pan and the jar. Simmer the jar until the beeswax is completely melted.

3 Remove from heat. Whisk until creamy and ingredients are completely incorporated. A hand blender is ideal for this step. Let cool until the cream can be handled.

4 Using a spatula, move the cream to a clean jar or storage container with a lid. Use within 60 days.

Notes

1   "Eczema," National Eczema Association, https://nationaleczema. org/ eczema.

THE "NO POO" SHAMPOO REVOLUTION

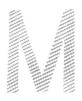any people looking to live a healthier, chemical-free, and more natural life have taken the challenge of rethinking the way they treat their hair. While the "no poo" shampoo movement has a lot of variations and room to customize what is best for your hair, all "no poo" solutions have one thing in common: never buying shampoo again. Some people using this philosophy try to limit the number of times they use natural shampoos to once a week or less, but this is not necessary. Although the shampoos in this book can be used often, Kirsten recommends washing your hair no more than twice a week.

If you type "no-poo shampoo" into an online search

engine, you will find many stories of people who have successfully made the switch—men, women, children, skeptics, whole families. Some people choose to take their hair through a "detox" by stripping the harsh chemicals in commercial shampoos from their hair. This detox period means that for a few weeks, your hair will become greasy and messy, but if you stick with it, the texture of your hair will change. This has worked successfully for people with long hair and short hair.

For those who desire to change their hair care habits but are concerned by a "detox" period of greasy, messy hair, we suggest using Honey Wet Shampoo for Oily Hair (see page 36), following the additional directions listed under that recipe. This will ease the transition.

For Caleb, the journey to a new approach to shampoo was born of necessity. No matter what shampoo he used—cheap or expensive, traditional or environmentally friendly—the residue of the shampoo would slowly work its way out of his super-thick, naturally oily hair and into his eyes. The chemicals from the shampoo would leave his eyes stinging and burning without warning in the middle of day. It happened so frequently and was so painful that Caleb began to wonder if his eyes might become damaged by the chemicals over time—after all, the pain and stinging must have been his body's way of sending a message that these chemicals are not meant for the eyes.

If you want to try going chemical-free, how do you get started? Stop washing your hair with purchased shampoo. Instead, use one of the options listed in this chapter.

BAKING SODA WET SHAMPOO

This shampoo recipe is simple and quick to make, with natural ingredients. And you will love the way it smells!

1/2 teaspoon baking soda
2–3 drops jojoba oil or tea tree
  oil (to soften the scalp)

1/2 cup warm water

 Stir the ingredients together in a bowl.

 Apply to your wet hair while in the shower. Gently scrub the baking soda mixture into your hair and rinse with warm water.

ARROWROOT DRY SHAMPOO

In addition to being great for your hair, this option also leaves your hair smelling great!

1/2 teaspoon arrowroot powder (use this alone for light-colored hair)
1/4 teaspoon cocoa powder (add this to the arrowroot for dark hair only)

1/4 teaspoon cinnamon (add this to the arrowroot for red hair only)

 If using more than arrowroot powder, mix ingredients together in a bowl.

 Apply to your dry hair. Gently massage the mixture into your hair and scalp, then brush the powder out with a hairbrush.

HONEY WET SHAMPOO FOR NORMAL HAIR

We strongly suggest you use a vegetable glycerin for this recipe (and any recipes in this book calling for glycerin), available at any health food store, or online. At first glance, you might not think honey would be a great ingredient for shampoo, but you will be surprised how cleansing and gentle this shampoo is on your hair!

1/4 cup raw honey   *1/4 cup distilled water**
2 tablespoons glycerin

*Use distilled water because it lasts longer than tap water since all bacteria has been removed.

 Mix the ingredients together.

 Apply to your wet hair in the shower, gently massaging the solution into your hair before rinsing with warm water.

Tip: You can put this solution into a hand pump bottle to keep in the shower.

HONEY WET SHAMPOO FOR OILY HAIR

This is Kirsten's favorite homemade shampoo—and soon may be yours, too!

1/4 cup raw honey
2 tablespoons glycerin

1 tablespoon baking soda
1/2 cup distilled water

 Mix the ingredients together.

 Apply to your wet hair in the shower, gently massaging the solution into your hair before rinsing with warm water.

Tip: If you want to ease the transition from commercial shampoo to "no-poo shampoo," add 1 teaspoon of liquid castile soap to this recipe. Each time you make the shampoo, cut the liquid castile soap amount in half until you are no longer using it in the recipe.

HONEY FRANKINCENSE SHAMPOO

Considering the ingredients, this shampoo recipe is almost biblical!

1/4 cup raw honey
2 tablespoons glycerin
1 tablespoon baking soda
1 tablespoon citric acid
   powder, or 2 tablespoons
   lemon or lime juice (use only
   if you have light-colored
   hair, because this can
   lighten hair color naturally)

1/2 cup distilled water
1 drop frankincense oil, or 1
   drop lemongrass essential
   oil (omit if this oil makes
   your hair greasy)

 Mix the ingredients together and keep in a squeeze bottle in your shower to use as regular shampoo.

 Apply to your wet hair in the shower, gently massaging the solution into your hair before rinsing with warm water.

TWO-PART NATURAL BORAX SHAMPOO

Borax is a naturally occurring substance produced by the repeated evaporation of seasonal lakes, according to the 20 Mule Team Borax company website. Borax is naturally soapy and 99.5% pure. The 0.5% of impurities consists of naturally occurring trace minerals. "Once removed from the ground, it is washed, dried, and boxed for consumers," according to the company. "20 Mule Team Borax comes from California, where one of the world's largest deposits was discovered in 1913. Absolutely nothing is added. No phosphates, peroxides, chlorine, or other additive chemicals."

PART ONE:

1 tablespoon borax powder   *1 cup warm water*

PART TWO:

1 tablespoon citric acid   *1 cup warm water*

1.   Mix the Part One ingredients together. In a separate container, mix the Part Two ingredients together.

2.   Apply the Part One mixture to your wet hair in the shower, gently massaging the solution into your hair

before rinsing with warm water. This will get rid of all grease and dirt.

 To wash the borax residue out of your hair, follow up with a rinse of the Part Two mixture.

YUCCA ROOT POWDER SHAMPOO

Yucca soapweed is a desert plant that Caleb grows in his yard. Both the roots and leaves are naturally soapy and have been used by Native Americans for centuries. You can buy seeds for the yucca soapweed plant at SeedRenaissance.com. You can also buy yucca root powder in health food stores, sometimes in bulk powder form and sometimes in capsules.

1 teaspoon yucca root powder   **1 cup warm water**

Combine both ingredients in a bowl. Allow the root powder to sit in the warm water for a couple of minutes to soften and begin to dissolve before using.

Use immediately to wash hair.

YUCCA LEAF OR ROOT SHAMPOO

Yucca is a desert plant that Caleb has grown for many years in his backyard. Both the leaves and roots are naturally soapy.

1 green leaf-spear of yucca soapweed, chopped, or a 1-inch piece of thick, fresh root

1 cup warm water

 Chop the root or leaf into small pieces and blend with the water until soapy (approximately 20–30 seconds).

 Strain out the root or leaf fibers using a mesh strainer, a reusable straining cloth (available at SeedRenaissance.com), or cheesecloth. Use the liquid soap immediately or store in a squeeze bottle for several days.

CONDITIONER AND HAIR STYLING

APPLE CIDER VINEGAR CONDITIONER & DETANGLER SPRITZ

Apple Cider Vinegar has many uses, and this is just one of them. If you want to learn to make your own homemade, organic, perpetual apple cider vinegar from a starter, go to SeedRenaissance.com.

2 tablespoons apple cider
   vinegar*

1/2 cup water
1 drop essential oil (optional)

*If your hair is naturally oily, use distilled white vinegar instead of apple cider vinegar, because distilled white vinegar is more drying.

1   Pour the vinegar and water (and essential oil if desired) into a spray bottle and shake gently to mix.

2   Spray onto the tips of your hair, or spritz it onto your whole head while your hair is wet after your shower. Avoid the scalp. Spritz only lightly—no need to dampen the hair or scalp with the solution.

Tip: Adding your favorite essential oil will help cut the vinegar smell, but if you spritz just a small amount, the vinegar smell should disappear in a couple of minutes. Because vinegar has a pH of about 4, this spritz helps balance the pH of your hair, leaving it healthier and easier to manage. Adding essential oil may also make your hair slightly greasy.

SCALP TREATMENT OILS AND SALVES

ANY OF THE FOLLOWING OILS WILL HELP SOOTHE THE SCALP WHILE RELIEVING DANDRUFF AND ITCHING:

- PURE ARGAN OIL
- TEA TREE OIL
- COMFREY-INFUSED OIL (SEE PAGE 22)
- CALENDULA-INFUSED OIL (SEE PAGE 22)
- PEPPERMINT-INFUSED OIL OR ESSENTIAL OIL

TIP: BE SURE TO USE OIL, NOT SALVES, BECAUSE SALVES CONTAIN BEESWAX

DEEP CONDITIONER

If your hair is dry or damaged, massage coconut oil through your hair.

Coconut oil

1. Use only a small amount of oil—just enough to hydrate your hair. Start at the end of your hair and work toward the crown of your head.

2. If you have a dry scalp, rub the oil into your scalp, too. Cover your hair with a towel and let the oil sit for up to half an hour before washing it out with Two-Part Natural Borax Shampoo (see page 38) or Honey Frankincense Shampoo (see page 37).

HOMEMADE HAIRSPRAY

"This is one of those homemade options that is old and simple and has been around since my grandmother was young," says Kirsten. Sometimes the old favorites bear repeating for those who may not have been taught them.

1/2 cup warm water   *1 tablespoon granulated sugar*

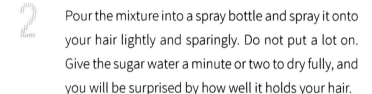

1. Stir the two ingredients together until the sugar has completely dissolved.

2. Pour the mixture into a spray bottle and spray it onto your hair lightly and sparingly. Do not put a lot on. Give the sugar water a minute or two to dry fully, and you will be surprised by how well it holds your hair.

Tip: If you live in a climate prone to rain, use this spray sparingly, because your hair may become sticky if you use too much of it.

HOMEMADE HAIR MOUSSE

Egg whites have been used throughout history for many things not related to cooking—they were even used by some of the world's most famous artists to make paint. In this profoundly simple recipe, you can use the beaten egg white as mousse to style your hair. Best of all, this mousse will, over time, give your hair a healthy shine!

1 egg white

Beat egg white to soft peaks.

Use just enough egg white mousse to achieve the look you are going for, then allow it a couple of minutes to dry completely.

"NEVER SNOTTY" HAIR GEL

"My son has something called 'Gorilla Snot Gel,' and he thinks it is so funny," says Kirsten. Clearly, the branding is aimed straight at young men, who, because of a natural lack of confidence that seems to be part of being a teen, often seem to be easily swayed by products promising instant masculinity and attention from young women. (In Caleb's opinion, these products often seem overpriced and overwhelming in their clear-the-room scents and seem to prey on the low self-esteem of some teens.)

1–2 teaspoons aloe vera gel

 Simply apply the aloe vera gel to your coif.

Tip: Beware that many products that claim to be "pure" or "100 percent" aloe vera gel actually contain many chemical ingredients. Read the labels before you buy—or better yet, grow your own aloe vera houseplant!

HARD LESSON LEARNED: THE IMPORTANCE OF LABELING HOMEMADE HERBAL PRODUCTS

I n two different instances, Kirsten's beloved husband, Steven, has unwittingly ingested things that looked like food but turned out to be one of Kirsten's herbal concoctions. Both stories are a humorous reminder about the serious issue of putting correct labels on all homemade products.

Kirsten once made some honey shampoo with several ingredients and put it in an empty honey container—and then absentmindedly left it sitting in the kitchen. Her husband, unaware that the honey had been turned into shampoo, came into the kitchen in the morning and put the homemade shampoo on his toast. "Something is wrong with this honey, honey!" he said. This turned out to be a funny story only because her husband was not harmed.

Another time, Kirsten was using hydrogen peroxide—a colorless, odorless liquid—for one of her homemade concoctions, and she had poured the liquid into a drinking glass for convenience. She left the glass on the kitchen table, and her husband mistook it for a glass of water and drank it. He said it burned all the way down. In this instance, too, her husband ended up OK but could not have been very pleased.

Whenever you create any kind of homemade product, always put a correct label on it immediately. It is important that the label contains a list of all ingredients in the product so that in case of accidental ingestion, you can call poison control and you will be able to tell them what has been ingested. Homemade products should be stored safely where they cannot be ingested by any member of the family—spouses, children, or pets. Ingredients like borax and hydrogen peroxide, while 100 percent natural and useful, should never be ingested. If someone in your family has accidentally ingested a homemade product, call poison control immediately.

AVOIDING TOXIC SHOCK SYNDROME WITH MENSTRUAL CUPS

Accrding to the US Centers for Disease Control, thousands of cases of toxic shock syndrome are diagnosed by doctors each year in the United States in connection with young girls using tampons.[1] The problem occurs when *Staphylococcus aureus* bacteria colonize in a menstrual tampon, producing chemicals that are toxic to the human body.[2]

According to the UK Tampax website, TSS "is a serious illness which can be fatal. It is caused by the toxins produced by the bacterium *Staphylococcus aureus* which is commonly found in the nose and vagina. TSS can occur in men, women and children. Approximately one-half of TSS cases occur in women and girls during their menstruation and this menstrual TSS is associated with tampon use. It is more likely to occur in teenage girls and women under 30 than in older women." Symptoms include a sudden high fever, vomiting, rash, fainting, peeling skin, diarrhea, sore throat, and muscle aches.[3] Because of concerns about TSS, there is a growing movement among women of all ages to use menstrual cups as an alternative to tampons. Kirsten was recommended menstrual cups long ago by a friend and again recently by her doctor.

Menstrual cups made of glass and silicone are sold under the brand names Diva Cup, Keeper Cup, Moon Cup, Lunette, and many others. The manufacturers tout these as being healthier for women and the environment.

"This changed my life as far as activity and not having TSS problems," says Kirsten. "I use a menstrual cup because there is no chance of toxic shock syndrome and there is no need to stop your activity. There is no restriction at all." One type of cup may be more comfortable than another for different women, but they all reduce cramping. The cups come in various sizes for younger girls or women who have had children. "It cuts down a lot on costs and on what ends up at the landfill," says Kirsten. "There are very good instructions available on the Internet on how to use it."

According to the manufacturers of one brand of menstrual cup, the average woman will use a staggering 11,000 tampons or pads in her lifetime.[4] The cost alone is a reason to consider a reusable menstrual cup. Even if it is not something you want to explore at this time, having a menstrual cup for emergencies, or in preparedness for unforeseen disasters or catastrophes, would be wise.

Notes

1   Rana A. Hajjeh et al., "Toxic shock syndrome in the United States: surveillance update, 1979–1996," Emerging Infectious Diseases 5, no. 6 (1999): 807–10.

2   "Toxic Shock Syndrome—TSS: Reducing the Risks," Tampax, http://www.tampax.co.uk/en-gb/foryourinfo/toxic-shock-syndrome-symptoms.aspx

3   Ibid.

4   Mooncup, http://www.mooncup.co.uk

AND FOR FUN . . . TWO HISTORIC COMPLEXION REMEDIES

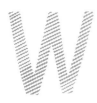e thought these were too fun to pass up, but we don't recommend trying these recipes.

MADAME VESTRIS'S COMPLEXION PASTE

he following is the recipe for the paste, by the use of which Madame Vestris is said to have preserved her beauty till very late in life. It is applied to the face on retiring for the night. The white of four eggs boiled in rose water, half an ounce of alum, half an ounce of oil of sweet almonds, beat the whole together until it assumes the consistence of a paste."[1]

QUEEN BESS'S COMPLEXION WASH

The following recipe has been handed down from the time of Queen Elizabeth. Its daily use preserved the beauty of her complexion to extreme old age. Into a phial place one drachm of Benzoin gum in powder, the same quantity of grated nutmeg, and about six drops of the essence of orange blossoms; then fill up the bottle with a wine-glassfull of the finest sherry. Shake the ingredients every day for a week, then mix the whole with a pint of orange-flower water; strain through fine muslin, and the 'Lait Virginal' is finished. The face is to be bathed with it night and morning."[2]

Notes

1   *Alvin Wood Chase and William Wesley Cook,* Dr. Chase's Recipes or Information for Everybody *(Stanton and Van Vliet Co. Publishers, 1920).*

2   *Ibid.*

FREE OFFER: TO GET A FREE PACKAGE OF HERB SEEDS, CLICK ON THE "FREE OFFERS" TAB AT SEEDRENAISSANCE.COM.

ABOUT THE AUTHORS

Kirsten Skirvin was born and raised in southern California. She spent a large part of her youth backpacking and camping with her family. Her father was the first to teach her the amazing properties of the plants around her. After receiving her BS in psychology from Brigham Young University, she continued spending time in the wild. She received her Master Herbalist degree from the School of Natural Healing in 2005 and has taught many herbal classes throughout the years. She hopes to inspire others to plant and harvest their own herbal medicines. She spends her time making tinctures, spinning wool, and dabbling in other old world crafts. She and her husband currently reside in Utah with their seven children.

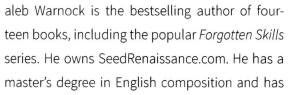

aleb Warnock is the bestselling author of fourteen books, including the popular *Forgotten Skills* series. He owns SeedRenaissance.com. He has a master's degree in English composition and has won more than two dozen awards for writing. Together with Kirsten Skirvin, he coauthored the book *Forgotten Skills of Backyard Herbal Healing and Family Health*. You can find all the episodes of Forgotten Skills Radio with Caleb Warnock at www.MormonHippie.com/category/forgotten-skills-radio/. Sign up for Caleb's newsletter on the bottom left-hand corner of SeedRenaissance.com. Caleb and his wife, Charmayne, live on the bench of the Rocky Mountains.

ABOUT FAMILIUS

Welcome to a place where mothers are celebrated, not compared. Where heart is at the center of our families, and family at the center of our homes. Where boo boos are still kissed, cake beaters are still licked, and mistakes are still okay. Welcome to a place where books—and family—are beautiful. Familius: a book publisher dedicated to helping families be happy.

VISIT OUR WEBSITE: WWW.FAMILIUS.COM

Our website is a different kind of place. Get inspired, read articles, discover books, watch videos, connect with our family experts, download books and apps and audiobooks, and along the way, discover how values and happy family life go together.

JOIN OUR FAMILY

There are lots of ways to connect with us! Subscribe to our newsletters at www.familius.com to receive uplifting daily inspiration, essays from our Pater Familius, a free ebook every month, and the first word on special discounts and Familius news.

BECOME AN EXPERT

Familius authors and other established writers interested in helping families be happy are invited to join our family and contribute online content. If you have something important to say on the family, join our expert community by applying at:

www.familius.com/apply-to-become-a-familius-expert

GET BULK DISCOUNTS

If you feel a few friends and family might benefit from what you've read, let us know and we'll be happy to provide you with quantity discounts. Simply email us at specialorders@familius.com.

Website: www.familius.com
Facebook: www.facebook.com/paterfamilius
Twitter: @familiustalk, @paterfamilius1
Pinterest: www.pinterest.com/familius

THE MOST IMPORTANT WORK YOU EVER DO WILL BE WITHIN THE WALLS OF YOUR OWN HOME.

CPSIA information can be obtained
at www.ICGtesting.com
Printed in the USA
FSOW01n1609050416
18857FS